Tooley's

60-Second

Pain

Turn Down

Easy Chronic Pain Relief in 1-Minute
Using Your Mind

DUNCAN TOOLEY, CHI

Mind Trainer & Medical Hypnotherapist

Do-It-Yourself Pain Relief Resources
You Deserve to Feel GREAT!
I know you can easily adjust to feel great!

Additional tools available at:
feelgreat.duncantooley.com

- Mantra Reminder Cards
- Tooley 60-Second Turn Down Process
- Acupressure Tapping Points Diagram
- Tune Your Mindset Worksheet
- My Comfort Control Chart
- Positive Words That Will Enrich Your Mind & Soul
- Positive Affirmation List
- Feel Great Word Search Puzzle
- List of Medical Issues Benefiting from Hypnosis
- Sunrise Mandala Image
- Mandala Coloring Book

Email Contact: *duncan@duncantooley.com*
Call **310-832-0830 for hypnosis at-a-distance options**
Also see artworks by the author at: **art.duncantooley.com.com,**
and more hypnosis information at: *hypnosis.duncantooley.com*

This little book is your
PAIN RELIEF ANSWER!

"It's almost like a magic spell. I have no pain. I have my old life back, able to do everything I want pain-free." -- Rebecca Harris"

It was amazing! Duncan's process stopped my serious pain from six surgeries and a fused ankle." -- Shelley Fine

"Ten years of chronic pain instantly decreased dramatically. I stopped taking six Codeine pills a day." -- Jane Smolens

"Duncan Tooley taught me how to turn off the pain, calm the itching, and make my red skin bumps disappear. . . I had no idea that I could easily have control over my pain." -- Dina Wiley

"Duncan Tooley shows that you can become pain free. You don't have you don't have to struggle with pain for years, or accept being in pain as a normal way of life." -- Dr. Leyla Ali, Pharmacist and Author of *Off Balance, The American Way of Health, A Pharmacist's Perspective on Why Drugs Don't Work.*

"If you want relief, this book is a must read." -- Shelley Stockwell Nicholas, PhD, President, International Hypnosis Federation.

"Duncan Tooley generously shares how to communicate with pain, and then use your will, intention, and mind to repair and restore. Almost too simple and effective to be believed! It just works!" -- Dr. Aviva Boxer, OMD, (DrAvivaBoxer.com) "Restoring radiant vitality, resilience and stamina without an expiration date."

"When I had my back incident, I could not get up off the floor until I used Tooley's 60-second Turn Down technique" -- Glen Michael

Tooley Transformation Training Publications
2742 San Ramon Drive
Rancho Palos Verdes, CA 90275
310-832-0830   email: FeelGreat@duncantooley.com

FAIR USE NOTICE

DISCLOSURE

This book is for educational purposes and does not pretend to constitute the practice of medicine in any way. The techniques presented here are stand-alone and legal adjunct health-care, help-care wellness approaches and not the exclusive domain of any licensed healing arts profession. Many of the techniques presented are extremely popular because of their profound positive results. The author and publisher expressly disclaim responsibility for any adverse effects arising from the use, misuse, non-use, or application of the information contained in this book. You are a unique individual in your expression of mind-body-spirit. Use what is appropriate for you.

ACKNOWLEDGEMENTS

Thanks to Dr. Richard Steiner, Dr. Marita Pall, Dr. Leyla Ali, Janet Stanakis, Eva Margueriette, my family, and numerous friends for encouragement and editorial assistance. Special thanks to Dr. Shelley Stockwell-Nicholas, my teacher, mentor, coach, and friend in hypnosis and publishing. Acupressure diagram based on www.thetappingsolution.com. Artwork by the author with mandala images provided by Shelley Stockwell and students in my creative mandala classes.

DEDICATION

This book is dedicated to YOU,
dear reader.
I wrote this for you and those you love.

As a Mind Trainer and
Medical Hypnosis Instructor,
I know that this simple process,
plus the natural power
of your body-mind-spirit,
will transform your life
so you feel great.

Duncan

Contents

▶Introduction . . . About Pain 1

▶Tooley 60-Second PAIN Turn Down 7

▶Appendix
A1. Affirmations 15
A2. Laughter 21
A3. Mind-Body-Spirit Model 23
A4. Mind Principles 33
A5. Medical Benefits of Hypnosis 37
A6. Hypnosis Myths Busted 51

▶About The Author 61

▶Do-It-Yourself Pain Relief Resources 63

Introduction

About **Pain**

The REIGN of PAIN is mainly in the BRAIN!

Fundamental Truth

Your brain cannot tell the difference between your perception of an experience and the actual physical experience. What you tell your mind, your mind believes.

Your mind gets input from three sources:
- Your senses
- Your memory
- Your imagination

Your mind treats the information from all three inputs equally. Your mind cannot tell the difference between senses, memory, and imagination.

You have the power to direct your imagination any way you choose. As a result, you are able to take control of the effects of your memory and your senses with your imagination and turn off pain. It is this power of your imagination, working with the physiology of your body, that is the basis for the techniques in this book.

This book is for you if you experience any kind of pain. You don't have to own the pain, so I avoid calling any discomfort "your" pain.

Physiology of Your Nervous System

The nervous system of your body is composed of the central nervous system (the brain and spinal cord), the peripheral nervous system (the sensory and motor neurons), and the autonomic nervous system (which regulates body processes such as digestion and heart rate). The processes in this book will assist you to train your brain to interpret information from your nervous system in the way that makes you feel great!

Brain and Pain

Your brain is the endpoint of the relay system that is the pain network. When a peripheral nerve fires, the signal is passed to the nerves in the spinal cord. The information is processed there and passed to the brain stem. Part of the spinal cord processing may involve firing a motor nerve cell to stimulate a muscle contraction to move the affected area away from the pain source.

The information passed to the brain stem goes to the mid-brain region. From there it is analyzed and may be sent to the cortical brain region, specifically that area that has come to be known as the brain's *pain center*. It is at that point that you *feel* the pain.

Pain As Interpretation

Something is happening in the body, and your brain applies meaning and triggers emotion to interpret what is going on. This means that if your brain did not interpret, then there would be no pain! The pain occurs only after the circuit is completed by the brain's interpretation of the signal.

Consider how many times you may have cut yourself without realizing it. Perhaps it was a paper edge or a sharp blade you were using. Most likely it did not hurt until you *saw* the blood, possibly minutes or more after the cut actually happened! This shows your brain's role in interpreting what it believes *should be* pain.

How to Stop Pain?

The three methods for stopping the sensation of pain all focus around preventing the nerve stimulation signal from reaching that bundle of brain neurons that is identified as the pain center:

1. **Stop the nerve stimulation at its source.** This stops the peripheral nerve cells from firing. In its simplest form this is something like: "Take your hand out of the fire!"

   Local anesthetics are also in this category. They chemically bind to nerve cells and prevent them from producing nerve signals.

2. **Block the signal from reaching the brain.** Neurons sensitive to vibration, temperature, and pressure transmit at a faster rate than pain neurons. Therefore, it is possible to flood the neural pathway with other nerve sensations so that the pain signal gets blocked or overpowered.

   When you instinctively rub a painful area or apply heat or cold to "relieve" the pain, what you are doing is blocking the pain signal from reaching your brain by flooding the neural relay system with other information. (Epidural injections and nerve blocks also operate by this method of blocking the pain signal from reaching your brain. They are listed here for information and not as a recommendation).

3. **Prevent the signal from reaching the pain center.** Even though the nerve signal has arrived in your brain, you do not feel the sensation of discomfort until your brain processes it and sends it to the *pain center*. This method prevents the signal from being *interpreted* as pain by stimulating other parts of your brain instead of the pain center. Most of the techniques in this book work like this.

Call Pain by Its Proper Name!

There is nothing either good or bad, but thinking makes it so. - Hamlet 2, 2

Pain is mostly named from a time perspective: *acute,* short term, and *chronic,* long term. Sometimes we call pain *good pain* or *bad pain.* However, from your brain's perspective, what counts is the purpose and intelligence conveyed by the discomfort. From your brain's point of view, pain is either *informational* or *nuisance.*

Informational pain signals that something is not as it should be and needs attention. Informational pain is giving your mind, INFORMATION. Listening to your body provides information about the cause of discomfort, so that you can choose an appropriate response.

Nuisance pain is just that, a useless nuisance. Nuisance pain adds no value by its continuation after you have taken whatever measures you can to remedy what the informational pain was reporting. Not only does this pain have no value, it often adds debilitating stress.

Use the techniques in this book to relieve *nuisance* pain. If discomfort continues to get your attention, the discomfort you experience may still be *informational,* calling you to learn more from your body. Begin now to learn to discern from the Tooley 60-Second Turn Down technique in this book what is *informational pain* and what is *nuisance pain* for you.

Story: My client, Glen, suffered a ruptured vertebra disc while alone at work. He couldn't get off the floor until he used my *60-Second Turn Down* method (Chapter 2). Later he told me it would have been impossible to drive to the hospital had he not used that method to lower his experience of pain.

Analysis: Since Glen had accepted the informational value of the pain, ("Something in my back needs attention!"), and had decided upon a remedial action ("Get to the hospital!"), it was appropriate to convert his *informational* pain experience into a *nuisance* pain that he could turn off. Even though nothing about the firing of his neurons had changed, he transformed his discomfort into a *nuisance* by his remedial action and his decision to ignore the pain. Notice that the difference between *informational* and *nuisance* pain is in your brain, not in the pain source.

My Story: My right knee was screaming when I walked, so I went to my physician to have it checked. I used that *informational* pain to seek the appropriate remedial action, if any. An MRI revealed the jagged edge of a torn meniscus. The doctor recommended surgery to trim off the jagged edge.

When I decided not to do the surgery, that decision effectively converted my *informational* pain to *nuisance* discomfort. The original pain had done its job and now it was just a nuisance that I could ignore. I used the *Affirmations* method (Chapter 11) on my knee. Since then it has been very comfortable, only reminding me of its presence after *extreme* activity.

Caution!

Just because you learn the methods to interpret a discomfort as a nuisance and remove it from your perception doesn't mean that this is the best thing for you to do. You must make the personal decision about what is in your best interest in each case. Only you know what is normal and OK for your body to endure. Be careful; be safe; listen to your body's information. Decide wisely when to consider discomfort a nuisance and turn it off via the methods in this book, and when to consider it information that you must continue to investigate.

Many athletes turn off or ignore informational pain. Often they suffer permanent injuries as a result.

> *Story:* Famous baseball player Lou Gehrig played 2,130 consecutive baseball games despite broken fingers. When Gehrig's hands were X-rayed late in his career, doctors spotted 17 different fractures that had *healed* while Gehrig continued to play. Gehrig had decided to ignore, 17 times, the informational pain from his broken fingers. He decided to consider the pain as nuisance pain and used his mind to ignore it.

Say Your Mantra Often:

> *"I discern whether my discomfort is **Informational** or **Nuisance**.*
> *If **Informational**, I listen and take appropriate action.*
> *If **Nuisance**, I turn it off."*

> *Extra:* Print six reminder cards with your mantra from the book extras website: *www.feelgreat.duncantooley.com*

~◻~◻~◻~

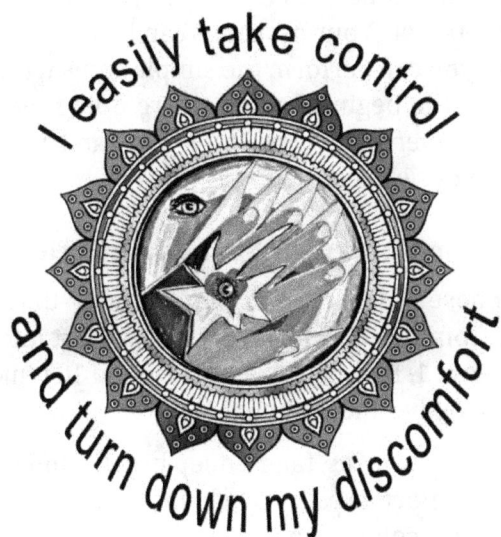

I easily take control and turn down my discomfort

Tooley's **60-Second Pain Turn Down**

About Tooley 60-Second Turn Down

This technique uses the power of your imagination. It is quick, simple, easy to remember, and very effective. Your subconscious mind accepts imagination in the same way that your subconscious accepts the information coming in through your senses. Nearly everyone experiences significant relief with this turn-down process. Consider it your first line of offense for feeling better. At least 50% pain reduction is usual, and many achieve 100% removal of discomfort.

If you have someone who can assist you for the first time, that's even better. Your assistant can lead you through the process so you can perform the simple steps with your eyes closed from the beginning. If you are doing the technique by yourself, memorize the steps first and then perform them with your eyes closed.

Steps to Use Tooley 60-Second Turn Down

1. Choose only one area of your body that is causing discomfort. Measure your discomfort intensity on a scale of 1-10, where 1 is very low and 10 is most intense. Remember the number.

2. Close your eyes, take a deep breath, and imagine the discomfort area as a shape, any shape. Give the shape a color (or a smell if you prefer).

3. Change the shape to some other shape then change the color (or smell) to another color (or smell). Change the shape and color slowly two more times.

4. Imagine a round volume control knob with the numbers 0 through 11 around the edge. Place the knob on top of your final shape, with the arrow pointing to the number of your discomfort level from the first step.

5. Reach in and grab the knob and slowly turn it *UP* one number, making the pain intensity higher than your starting number, only for a moment. When you feel your discomfort increase, turn the control back down to where you started.

6. Slowly turn the knob down one number at a time, pausing on each number until the discomfort

decreases on each step down. You can stop wherever you choose, or you can continue to turn the knob and decrease the discomfort all the way down to zero.

Congratulations! That was great! Good job!

Notice how comfortable you feel! Amazing, isn't it! You have taken control and now you feel much better! You used your mind to control your body! You can always do this exercise to feel great!

Why this technique works

If pain happens to you, you can easily feel like a victim. In the *Tooley 60-Second Turn Down* process, you gradually take control back from pain and restore your power as you move from "victim" to "controller." First you take artistic control with the shape and color. Then you take intensity control with the "volume" knob adjustments.

PAIN, of itself, never really had any power. Whatever power pain seemed to have, you gave to it by surrendering *your* power over interpretation of what is happening in your body. With this turn-down process you affirm your power to interpret body sensations however you choose! You re-frame your experience from "victim" of discomfort to being a powerful "controller" of how you feel.

> *Story:* When I was a presenter at a health fair, I used the 60-Second Turn Down technique with a man who said his pain level was a "10." At the end of the process his pain level was "0"! He called me a "Miracle Worker." I reminded him that HE is the miracle worker because he used the power of his mind to change his perception of pain. I assisted by supplying the technique that showed him how to do it.

Story: At a different wellness event, a woman came up to me on crutches. "I have a very painful heel spur," she said. When I asked her, "Would you like to reduce the pain level?" she answered "Yes, my pain level is 10." I instructed her to sit down and then used the *60-Second Turn Down* technique with her. After she opened her eyes and stood up, she exclaimed "The pain is gone! I can't believe it!" She went off carrying her crutches, looking for her husband to tell him.

Story: A client to whom I had taught the *60-Second Turn Down* technique had a dramatic back pain episode while alone at work. He later told me, "Using your technique allowed me to turn down my pain level enough so I could drive myself to the hospital. Before I used it, I was unable to get up off the floor."

Story: A participant in a cancer support services meeting told me she was suffering with pain. I used my *60-Second Turn Down* technique after the meeting with her. When I saw her a month later, she told me that she had successfully used the process many times for relief. She prevailed upon the administration of the cancer support center to add instruction about this technique to their curriculum of services.

Pro-Tip: If you are assisting someone in decreasing their discomfort by reading the instructions to them, be certain to include these important steps:

• Increase the pain level by turning the control knob *UP* one digit. This is the key empowering step because once a person experiences that the pain actually increases when they turn the knob up (and they will experience an increase!), they realize that they are able to control the discomfort sensation. The increase becomes the powerful convincer that they can decrease pain by turning the knob down!

• Offer to stop at intensity level 3, and level 2, and level 1. Initially the person you are assisting may not be able to believe that they can turn pain down lower than a level 3 or 2 or 1. The option of stopping at one of these levels permits the person to solidify the experience of lowering discomfort without violating their core beliefs. With subsequent uses they may be able to go lower.

Most who go for turning their discomfort down to level "0" (no discomfort) succeed in reaching it. They achieve level zero because, as they feel the discomfort decrease, they release any doubt of their ability to reach level zero. The power of their belief that they are in control makes complete relief a reality for them.

Extra: Get the *Tooley 60-Second Turn Down* process written as a script to be used with another person. Get a friend to use it with you. Download and print from the book extras website: *www.feelgreat.duncantooley.com*

~◻~◻~◻~

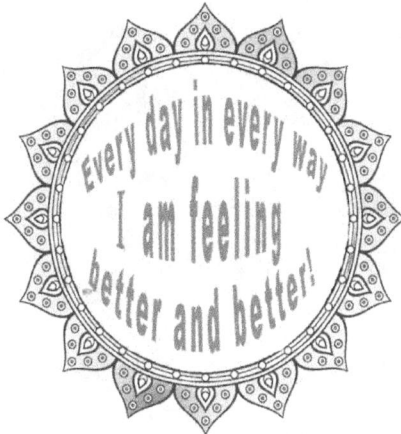

▶Appendix
Related Pain Relief Information

A1. Affirmations 15

A2. Laughter 21

A3. Mind-Body-Spirit Model 23

A4. Mind Principles 33

A5. Medical Benefits of Hypnosis 37

A6. Hypnosis Myths Busted 51

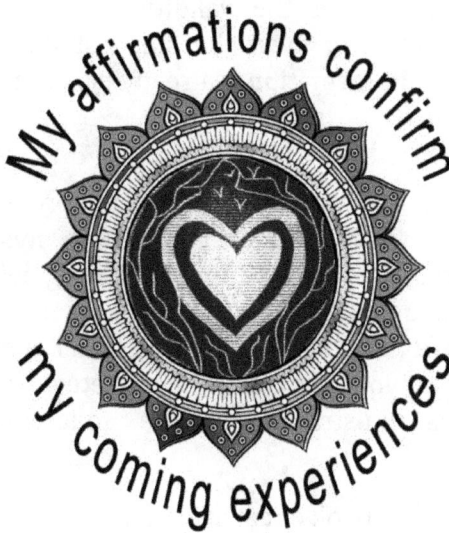

My affirmations confirm my coming experiences

Affirmations

About Affirmations

Affirmations are short messages to your subconscious for the purpose of strengthening a belief and prompting your subconscious to act in alignment with that belief. They are instructions to yourself about what you desire to believe to be true. The instruction has the effect of becoming absolutely true in every sense such that you *know* and *experience* its truth.

The goal of using affirmations is to move from *desiring* to *believing,* to *knowing with absolute certainty,* the truth stated in the affirmation. The goal is that there is not the slightest doubt about the validity of that truth. That certainty, absence of even the smallest doubt, is what guarantees your affirmation is already becoming reality!

Belief vs. Certainty

The power of affirmations is in the difference between belief and certainty. I once considered myself a very religious person and thought that my strong belief was the highest form of faith. Then I learned that belief is not enough! There is a tiny *lie* hidden in be*lie*f, a small doubt that can hold you back from complete certainty. The difference is illustrated by the following thought experiment:

Imagine holding a book out at arm's length and ask yourself "What will happen when I release it?" You won't say "I BELIEVE the book will hit the floor." I predict you will say something like: "The book will hit the floor."

And if questioned about your certainty of that result, you would say something like, "I KNOW it will hit the floor. I am certain it will hit the floor. I have not the slightest doubt that it will hit the floor."

The book falls because it obeys the Law of Gravity, which states: "Objects with physical mass attract each other." The earth pulls on a book with the same force that the book pulls on the earth. The book moves more toward the earth because its small mass moves more easily than the much larger mass of the earth. The force of attraction is the same however.

Every particle in the universe attracts every other particle. Water molecules attract the moon as strongly as the moon attracts the ocean's water molecules. The water molecules move upward and result in high tides without moving the moon out of its orbit.

Law of Attraction

The Law of Gravity is a subset of the general Law of Attraction. The attraction effect applies not just to objects with mass, but to all things. The Law applies to people being attracted to each other, to circumstances, to emotions, and to events. And, yes, the Law even applies to P@#$ (See Positive Self-Talk steps). Your thoughts attract more thoughts of comfort or discomfort, whichever you choose!

Some proverbs you may already know summarize the Law of Attraction's effects:

- *"Birds of a feather flock together."*
- *"What goes around comes around."*
- *"What you think about, comes about!"*
- *"What you think about (believe & tell yourself) is what you get (is attracted to you). "*

The Law of Attraction is always working whether we acknowledge the Law or not. Affirmations work with the Law of Attraction to get the relief we desire.

Steps to Use Affirmations for Relief
Step 1. Compose Your Affirmations.
- Use short, simple, easily repeatable declarative sentences.
- Use the present tense (no futures or potentials).
- Use only positive words (no form of negatives).
- Use only words of things you desire (no mention of things you don't want; for example, instead of "I am pain-free," use "I feel great!").

- Make your affirmation about you (not about other people, events, circumstances, or things).
- Use strong, emotional words, with *juice* or power (*beautiful, fantastic, awesome,* and *magnificent* are more powerful than *good*).
- Conclude with: "I am grateful that this or something better, is manifesting for me right now!"

Step 2. Use Proven Relief & Comfort Affirmations.

Affirmations that end discomfort and increase comfort and well-being that have proven their value with clients over the years are listed below. Most were gleaned from the writings of Shelley Stockwell-Nicholas, PhD.

- I feel GREAT!
- My life is a celebration.
- Everything I do allows me to enjoy my life more and more.
- I am healthy.
- My positive thoughts create my healthy body.
- My body is my perfect friend. I take care of my body.
- I am fully in tune with my body.
- I exercise and eat only healthy foods.
- I control my body with my mind.
- I give my body the "OK" to heal itself.
- I command my body to repair and renew itself now!
- I forgive myself for any mistakes I have made.
- In this moment I am cleansed.
- I learn from the past and then let the past go.
- I am joy.
- In this NOW moment I am happy, comfortable, and radiant.

Appendix 1. Affirmations

- As I breathe, every nerve, ligament, muscle, bone, fiber, and organ of my body comes into balance.
- The creative force within me heals me and keeps me well!
- All my body functions work perfectly and I know it!
- I feel terrific!
- Every little cell in my body is *happy* and *well!*"

Step 3. Make the Affirmations Part of Your Daily Life.
- Say them often. Write them. Post them where you see them. Chant them.
- Record them with feeling and listen to your recording often.
- Say or play them as you fall asleep at night and first thing upon awakening.
- Trust, allow, accept, believe, and *know* that they are already working for you!

Step 4. Repeat, Repeat, Repeat.
Determine your favorite affirmations and write them on six index cards. Place one card on your vanity mirror, refrigerator, car dashboard, computer monitor, night table, and in your wallet or purse. Say your affirmations from the card every time you see it. The one on your night table is the reminder to say your affirmations as you fall asleep and first thing upon awakening because these are the two most powerful times to do so.

Extra: Get a great list of affirmations at the book extras site: *www.feelgreat.duncantooley.com.*

~◻~◻~◻~

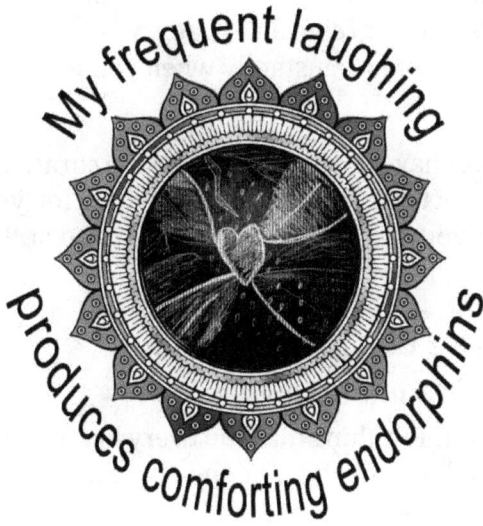

My frequent laughing produces comforting endorphins

Laughter

About Laughter

Laughter is the quickest, least expensive, always-available discomfort reliever. Your brain is a pharmaceutical chemical factory that produces endorphins when you laugh. Endorphins are a class of chemicals whose name is derived from "endogenous morphine," which means morphine produced by the body.

Make laughing work for you right now by searching your memory for the funniest thing that you ever heard or saw or did. When you retrieve it, have a good laugh! Then refile that memory in your brain's database under the category "instant discomfort reliever." That way you will be able to retrieve that memory instantly when you next want to feel better.

Many studies have been produced on the curative and pain-relieving effects of laughter. Try laughter for yourself. I'll wager that you can't have a good laugh and still feel like a victim of discomfort.

Steps to Use Laughter for Relief

Step 1. Use Your Memory.
Recall the funniest thing that you every heard or saw or did. Have a good laugh over it, and then repeat.

Step 2. Use the Laugh Formula.
A way to get a good laugh going is to use the formula that laughing is just the "H" sound on the front of each of the vowels:

> *"Ha, ha, ha, ha, ha, ha, ha!"*
> *"He, he, he, he, he, he, he!"*
> *"Hi, hi, hi, hi, hi, hi, hi!"*
> *"Ho, ho, ho, ho, ho, ho, ho!"*
> *"Hu, hu, hu, hu, hu, hu, hu!"*
> *"Isn't that funny?"*

Step 3. Use the Internet.
Find and watch videos of funny things that make you laugh, like compilations of dogs or cats doing astounding tricks. Search for and watch the 50 funniest YouTube videos.

~ ❑ ~ ❑ ~ ❑ ~

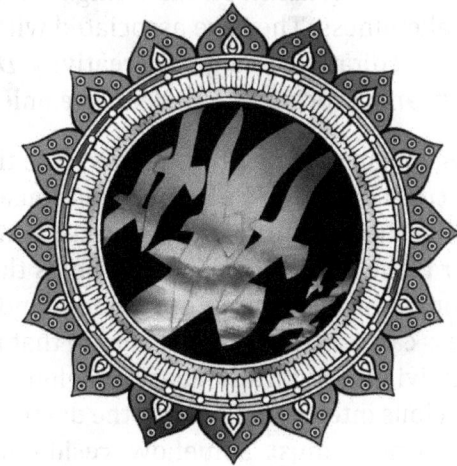

Mind-Body-Spirit Model

What is Mind?

Mind and brain are not the same. We don't understand the role the brain plays in consciousness. We can measure the existence of thoughts (and aspects of consciousness) in the brain, and we can use the predominant frequency of brain waves to determine the level of consciousness. Brain activity of *beta* waves above 13 hertz (cycles per second) indicate high consciousness (alertness, concentration, anticipation). *Alpha* waves from 7 hertz to 13 hertz are associated with tranquil, relaxed wakefulness. This is the brain wave pattern during meditation. *Theta* waves from 4 hertz to 7 hertz are considered the twilight state between sleep and wakefulness. They are associated with hypnosis, dreams, deep meditation, and great creativity. *Delta* waves below-4 hertz are associated with deep dreamless sleep.

What is consciousness? The brain seems to be the physical device for consciousness but not consciousness itself, somewhat like the memory chip in a cell phone or audio music player is the physical device that holds the song, but is not the song. The real gap in our understanding is how consciousness can continue after the organ that is the brain is no longer living. Practically every religion affirms that there is conscious intelligent life after the death of the body. That consciousness must somehow reside beyond the physical limits of the brain.

The common word used to capture this fact is MIND, defined as "That element of a person that enables them to be aware of the world and their experiences, to think, and to feel; the faculty of consciousness and thought."

No one understands everything about how the mind works. Philosophers have speculated for centuries about the mind and consciousness. Scientists believe they are learning more each year, especially since they can monitor activity in certain parts of the brain in real time and relate that to mental activity associated with consciousness. Allusions to consciousness fill poetry, philosophy, religion books, and Shakespeare's plays. Yet consciousness is still a mystery as to how it all works in us. My clients find the "computer model" as an aid to their understanding.

Computer Model of Mind

Computer engineers were very shrewd; they designed computers to be very much like us. When you look at a desktop computer the first thing that you see is the hardware: the screen, keyboard, mouse, printer, and speakers. These are all devices to get the information into or out of the computer. Notice that each of these is connected to the central processing unit, or CPU, with electrical cables. This is like our body with its five senses all connected to our CPU, our brain, by the electrical cables that form our nervous system. Our senses are what get our information into and out of our brain, our central processor.

But what makes the computer really function and do useful work, of course, is the software. There are always two levels of software in every computer. The most obvious level is called the application software. This software is designed to get a specific task accomplished. It is where the works gets done. Typical application software programs are word processor, email, web browser, and spreadsheets. As the size of computers shrank to the size of smart phones, the name of application software shrank to "apps." The apps on your smart phone are today's application software programs on your pocket computer.

Conscience Mind Is Like Application Software

Your conscious mind where you do your work, your rational thought, your analyzing, computation, language, and planning is very much like application software. This is the part of your mind that believes it is in control and makes decisions. It is where you exert willpower. It is that part of your mind that is at this moment pondering these concepts and the implications of the last sentence. It may even be suggesting that you reread three paragraphs for greater understanding!

Underneath the application software in every computer, there is always another level of software that is the operating system. The operating system's role is to make everything work together, handle the many common essential tasks for every application program, and keep the intricacies of program code hidden. The operating system handles the details to keep everything running smoothly so you can do your work without interruption or distraction. Even when your computer seems idle, there are dozens of programs running in the operating system.

Your Subconscious Is Your Operating System

You have an operating system, too. It's your subconscious mind. It runs your body, your reactions, your emotions, and your habits. A habit is like a program stored in your nervous system and controlled by your subconscious. Your interpretation of the signals from your body is a habit program running in your subconscious. This habit generates your awareness of comfort or discomfort.

Your Subconscious Programs

You have thousands of involuntary, automatic, thoughtless responses that take you through your day. When you feel discomfort on a finger from touching a plate that is too hot, you automatically pull your hand back without thinking about it until afterward. Your response was totally automatic; there was no conscious thought involved. These same types of triggered responses apply to thought patterns, emotions, and skills. These are like subroutines, small programs that get you through most of life's activities. Habits are like bigger, more complex programs. Amazing how clever those computer engineers were to design software that works like we do!

Your Subconscious Mind Runs Your Body

Yes, it's true! Your subconscious is controlling your body. Your conscious mind sometimes controls your skeletal muscles, as when you decide to stretch. If you consciously think about it, you can also control your breathing and your blinking; but if you don't think about these, they will continue without your conscious thought.

All the rest of your body's *automatic* processes, like blood pumping and oxygenation, digestion, wound healing, cell regeneration, waste collection, immune responses, and hundreds more, are not under your conscious control. They are under the control of your personal operating system, your subconscious mind. The medical profession calls this your autonomic nervous system. The neurons in the autonomic nervous system attach to your organs, and like the brain, are the physical support for the metaphysical activity of the mind that continues to keep your life force active within your body.

What does this computer program analogy mean for relief of your discomfort? It means that your goal becomes having one or more relief techniques for nuisance discomfort running automatically as a habit. The relief method is like a program upgrade for your subconscious. When you install your upgrade, you will have obtained relief without drugs. You will have trained your brain to feel great, perhaps without your conscious mind even noticing the program change!

Energy Source

Electricity from a battery or connection to the power grid is what powers a computer. What powers you? Stop reading for a few moments and consider how you answer this question. What powers you? How you answer this question depends on your culture, education, religious background, and life experiences. Whatever your answer, it is important because it is ultimately your source of power for overcoming the discomfort that you experience. Some call it soul or life-force or Spirit. What do YOU call your ultimate source of life energy?

Connectivity

A computer also needs a connection to other resources for software updates and information. That connectivity is through the Internet to all the resources on the worldwide web. That Internet connectivity also provides connectivity to other individuals via email, teleconferences, or interactive video. This connectivity is essential for modern computers, including mobile devices.

Connectivity to others and to resources has always been part of life, but because of technology, the flow is more obvious with our smart-phone in our hand frequently throughout the day. What is your connectivity for operating system upgrades, access to remote resources, communication with remote individuals, or even deceased loved ones? Some call it intuition; others admit to some psychic powers. What do you call YOUR connections?

The popular name for connectivity to the resources of all living things and metaphysical energy is the *Super-conscious mind*. It is what powers you, no matter what your belief system. It gives you life by connecting you to all other life in the universe, to all resources past, present, and future (timeless), and to the divine. Your super-conscious mind is your discomfort-relief connection to your life source and to the resources beyond the material.

Many call these two components of energizing life-force and connectivity by the term *spirit*. Therefore, it is common to speak of us humans as composed of body, mind, and spirit, just as your computer is composed of hardware, software, electricity, and network connection.

You are a complete being integrating Mind, Body, and Spirit. Your goal to end discomfort and feel great will include techniques that encompass each of these aspects of your being.

Hidden Auto-Programs

Your subconscious mind is the home for your habits. A habit is like a program stored in your nervous system and controlled by your subconscious. You love habits because they free your conscious mind. You send a repetitive activity down to your subconscious as a program (habit) that you can run whenever you need without requiring conscious thought or energy.

Tying Your Shoes

When you first learned how to tie your shoes, it took conscious concentration to learn the pattern and teach your finger muscles the routine. As you repeated it, it got easier and easier. Once you repeated it enough, it became a habit. What that means is that you sent the conscious pattern of finger movements down to your subconscious as a fixed program to be run anytime you needed it. All you have to do now is put on shoes with laces, and the next thing you know, they are tied without any conscious thought. Your *shoe-lace-tying* program was automatically invoked to automatically fire your neurons to move your fingers in the right pattern to execute the tied knot. Meanwhile, your conscious mind could have been thinking about anything, but most likely was thinking about where you were about to walk once your shoes were tied.

Walking

The same is true for walking. As an infant, you spent conscious energy over an extended period of time learning how to walk. You concentrated on firing neurons to move muscles in a coordinated pattern that imitated what you saw adults doing. You worked hard at it because you wanted to be able to move around as easily as you saw adults doing. Their encouragement motivated you to keep trying to get the pattern right even though you kept falling.

Finally you figured it out and wobbled your first steps. With more practice, your walking got smoother, but still required conscious effort. Then, eventually, it required less and less conscious thought as it became a routine program or habit.

Now everything about walking is so ingrained into your subconscious that it no longer requires conscious thought. Once you decide (with your conscious mind) that you want to walk some place, Your subconscious autopilot uses your stored program *walking* to handle all of the details of the right muscles to move at the right times. (Note: Walking is an exceedingly complex program incorporating feedback from the feet that influences the formulation of the next commands to move the leg and foot muscles. That complexity has hindered the development of *walking* robots).

Driving

Driving is probably the most complex physical habit that you have developed. When you first learned how to drive, it was difficult to simultaneously focus on all those details to do at the same time. Now they do not require conscious thought.

When the brake lights of the car in front of you light up, your foot automatically comes off the accelerator and onto the brake pedal without conscious thought. When you want to turn, you involuntarily turn on the turn signal. These, and many other actions, are now all part of the automatic habit-program you call *driving.*

You have probably experienced, more than once, arriving at your destination and not remembering any details of the trip. That's because your conscious mind was busy with other things while your subconscious drove the car for the entire trip, taking care of all the details automatically.

Pavlov

Ivan Pavlov was a Russian scientist who won the 1904 Nobel Prize in Physiology/Medicine for his research on the digestive system and involuntary reflex actions. Pavlov is most famous for his experiment of ringing a bell when he fed his dogs. After doing this for several days, he rang the bell without putting any food out. His dogs salivated at the sound of the bell. He did it again and again. They salivated again and again, even though there was no food.

This behavior pattern has come to be known as a *conditioned reflex.* You can also call it a *subconscious program*, or an *automatic reaction,* or a *thoughtless response.* In the dogs' experience databases, food and salivating were connected to the bell ringing. The ringing bell sound accessed the bell-ringing memory in the dogs' databases and activated the associated responses. Pavlov also studied involuntary reactions to stress and discomfort.

These conditioned reflexes from the database of prior experiences work similarly in humans. That means emotions and sensations of discomfort, grief, anger, sadness, or joy associated with prior experiences are automatically triggered by similar new circumstances in each of us; that means in me and in you! They are a type of habit.

Why is this illustration of habits, automatic subconscious programs, and conditioned reflexes, important? Its purpose is to help you grasp the very essential truth: your subconscious is running most of your life. Your conscious mind likes to think that it is in control. However, just like in your computer, there are many programs running in your operating system, in your subconscious, about which you are not aware. You can add more habits that will similarly perform automatically. Let relief be such a habit!

Make Your Relief Techniques a Habit

The impact of this for your comfort level is that your current interpretation of discomfort is running as a subconscious program, a habitual way of interpreting bodily sensations. The goal for your feel-great project is to have one or more relief techniques running automatically as a habit program for any nuisance discomfort. Then you will have converted discomfort to comfort without drugs by the power of your mind. (And perhaps it will have been so easy and automatic that you did not even notice!)

~□~□~□~

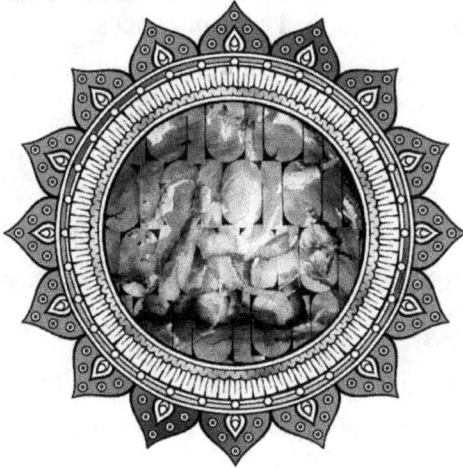

Mind Principles

How Your Mind Works

These principles of how the mind works are fundamental to the mind-over-body discomfort-relieving techniques in this book and the basis of my coaching. These formulations are from the teachings of Shelley Stockwell-Nicholas, PhD:

- You create your reality by your thoughts.
- You accept suggestions best in the language of your dominant sense.

- Your Self-Talk is hypnotizing you into a belief which affects everything.

- Thoughts are real things that radiate energy to affect people, events, and circumstances.

- Your mind affects your body and your body affects your mind.

- You remember and react best when strong emotion is attached.

- You imitate what you see your role models do.

- Change only occurs at the subconscious level.

- Change only occurs in the present moment.

- Readiness for change is half the change.

- You are single-minded. (You can only hold one thing in your mind at a time.)

- Habits run your life.

- What you affirm, you create.

- What you resist, you reinforce.

- What you insist, you resist.

- Your thoughts of anticipation initiate, create, and exaggerate.

- Energy flows where attention goes.

- Once you accept a belief, you find and emphasize what supports it, and you discount or ignore what contradicts your belief.

- You seek pleasure and avoid (or ignore) discomfort.

- *Try* implies failure. The harder you try, the more difficult it becomes.

- Imagination is more important than knowledge or logic.

- Your subconscious connects to the super-conscious Source of Ultimate Wisdom.

- Strong words work best.
- Your subconscious mind is literal. Use simple clear words and phrases.
- Repetition reinforces. Repetition plus repetition reinforces more than double.

Your mind is working all the time as the most complex machine in creation. The above is a short list of principles that describe some of the features of your mind that have been discovered. Apply these principles to help you discover the additional principles that are already working in your mind.

Pro-Tip: Understanding these principles and making them part of your belief system and actions will ease discomfort and promote feeling great. They will have a subtle, powerful effect on your entire life! A good approach is to take one principle at a time and turn it into a question about how it applies to you.

For example, based on the first three principles above:

- What reality am I creating in my life by my dominant thoughts?
- What is my strongest or dominant sense? Am I mostly visual, or do I learn and express through sounds, or smells, or feelings?
- What belief that isn't working for me is coming from my Self-Talk?

Ask the question(s) to yourself just before falling asleep and let your subconscious work on the answer while you sleep. You will awaken with more clarity. You may even dream about your question. Ask a different question each night, (unless your intuition suggests a repetition).

~◻~◻~◻~

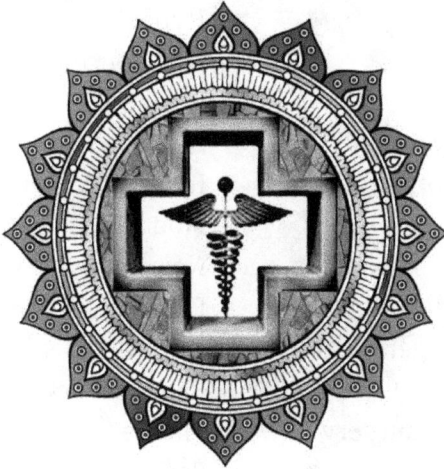

Medical Benefits of Hypnosis

Your subconscious mind runs your body. Therefore it follows that it should be possible to effect biological changes in your body by giving your subconscious mind instructions through hypnosis. Thousands of medical studies verify the truth of this logical conclusion.

Below is a partial list of the medical issues that benefit from hypnosis. Following the list is the abstract of each study that validated the hypnosis benefits.

Medical Issues Benefitting from Hypnosis-(partial list)

Acne

Addiction

Allergy

Alcoholism

Anesthesia for pain

Anesthesia for surgery

Asthma

Auto-immune disorders

Back pain (chronic)

Bleeding (surgery)

Boils (furuncles)

Breast cancer surgery

Cardiac surgery

Chemotherapy side effects

Childbirth

Constipation (chronic)

Dementia

Dermatitis

Eczema (neurodermatitis)

Face skin redness (rosacea)

Fibromyalgia

Hair loss (alopecia)

Hair pulling (trichotillomania)

Headaches (chronic)

Healing from injury

Healing from surgery

Hemophilia

Herpes

Hives (urticaria)

Hypertension

Impotence

Insomnia

Irritable bowel syndrome

Itching (pruritus)

Mouth-burning (glossodynia)

Neuralgia

Pain suppression

Panic attacks

Peptic ulcers

Phobias

Psoriasis

Psychogenic weakness

Seborrhea

Sedation (for surgery)

Skin - dry/scaly (ichthyosis)

Skin color loss (vitiligo)

Skin discoloration

Smoking cessation

Surgery recovery (all types)

Sweating excess (hyperhidrosis)

Thyroidectomies

Tinnitus (ringing in ears)

Urinary incontinence

Warts (verruca vulgaris)

Weight loss

Wound healing

Extra: Print this *Medical Issues Benefitting from Hypnosis* from the book extras website:
www.feelgreat.duncantooley.com

The Validating Studies for the Benefits:

Documented Results in Contemporary Medicine

A review study of over a hundred clinical studies of hypnosis for medical procedures documents that hypnosis is beneficial for allergy, anesthesia for pain, anesthesia for surgery, warts, dermatitis, irritable bowel syndrome, peptic ulcers, abdominal surgery, healing from injury or surgery, hemophilia, hypertension, headaches, childbirth, asthma, smoking cessation, fibromyalgia, impotence, and urinary incontinence. *"Many important trials reviewed have helped to establish the role of hypnosis in contemporary medicine. These trials have established the utility and efficacy of hypnosis for several medical conditions, either alone or as part of the treatment regimen."* (Cf. References, Study 13)

Success Rate 77 Percent for Drug Addiction

In a measure of 18 clients (15 for alcoholism or alcohol abuse, 2 cocaine addiction, and 1 for marijuana addiction), hypnosis showed a 77 percent success rate for at least a 1-year follow-up. (Cf. References, Study 14)

Hypnotherapy Bests Psychotherapy for Addicts.

In a comparative study of hypnotherapy and psychotherapy in the treatment of methadone addicts, significantly more methadone addicts quit with hypnosis. At six month follow up, 94% percent of the subjects who received hypnosis remained narcotic free. (Cf. References, Study 15)

Lost More Weight than 90% of Others & Kept It Off

Researchers analyzed 18 studies comparing a cognitive behavioral therapy such as relaxation training, guided imagery, self-monitoring, or goal setting with the same therapy supplemented by hypnosis. Those who received the hypnosis lost more weight than 90 percent of those not receiving hypnosis and maintained the weight loss two years after treatment ended. (Cf. References, Study 16)

Most Effective Way to Stop Smoking

Hypnosis is the most effective way of giving up smoking, according to the largest ever scientific comparison of ways of breaking the habit. A meta-analysis, statistically combining results of more than 600 studies of 72,000 people from America and Europe to compare various methods of quitting. On average, hypnosis was over three times as effective as nicotine replacement methods and 15 times as effective as trying to quit alone. (Cf. References, Study 17)

Guided Imagery Improves Cardiac Surgery Results

"Cardiac surgery patients who listened to a preoperative guided imagery surgical tape had significantly less pain, anxiety and two days shorter hospital stay." (Cf. References, Study 18)

Hypnosis Beneficial for Breast Cancer Surgeries

In a randomized study of 200 women undergoing surgery for breast cancer, those who received a brief hypnosis session before entering the operating room required less anesthesia and pain medication during surgery, and reported less pain, nausea, fatigue, and discomfort after surgery than women who did not receive hypnosis. The overall cost of surgery was also significantly less for women undergoing hypnosis. (Cf. References, Study 19)

Blood Flow Control during Surgery

In a trial with 93 spinal surgery patients at the University of California (Davis) Medical Center, those who received specific instructions about blood flow lost about half as much blood compared to the controls and a third group taught relaxation techniques. (Cf. References, Study 1)

Hypnosis Re-routes Signal Away from Pain Center

When hot plates were applied to volunteers, substantial pain was induced, and the live brain scan showed the signal routed to the pain center. Under hypnosis little or no pain was experienced and the brain scans revealed that the signal was routed to other parts of the brain, and not the pain center. *"It helps to dispel prejudice about hypnosis as a technique to manage pain because we can show an objective, measurable change in brain activity linked to a reduced perception of pain."* (Cf. References, Study 20)

Hypnosis Benefits Fibromyalgia

"In a controlled study, 40 patients with refractory fibromyalgia were randomly allocated to treatment with either hypnotherapy or physical therapy for 12 weeks with follow up at 24 weeks. Compared with the patients in the physical therapy group, the patients in the hypnotherapy group showed a significantly better outcome." (Cf. References, Study 21)

Hypnosis Improves or Cures Dermatologic Disorders

A comprehensive review of dermatology studies spanning 32 years that involved hypnosis concluded: *"A wide spectrum of dermatologic disorders may be improved or cured using hypnosis as an alternative or complementary therapy, including acne excoriee, alopecia areata, atopic dermatitis, congenital ichthyosiform erythroderma, dyshidrotic dermatitis, erythromelalgia, furuncles, glossodynia, herpes simplex, hyperhidrosis, ichthyosis vulgaris, lichen planus, neurodermatitis, nummular dermatitis, postherpetic neuralgia, pruritus, psoriasis, rosacea, trichotillomania, urticaria, verruca vulgaris, and vitiligo."* (Cf. References, Study 22)

Hypnosis Effective for Irritable Bowel Syndrome

"Previous research from the United Kingdom has shown hypnotherapy to be effective in the treatment of irritable bowel syndrome (IBS). The current study provides a systematic replication of this work in the United States." (Cf. References, Study 23)

Preoperative Suggestions Improve Abdominal Surgery Outcomes.

In a single-blind trial of abdominal surgery patients, to whom a 5 minute script was read preoperatively suggesting increased gastrointestinal motility after surgery, the suggestion group had significantly shorter ileus time (disruption of bowel movement) and was discharged two days earlier, with an estimated savings of $1200 (1993 dollars, Cf. References, Study 24)

Hypnosis for Dementia

Forensic psychologist, Dr. Simon Duff, (Univ. of Liverpool) compared the effects of hypnosis therapy with those of mainstream therapies for people suffering from dementia, and group therapy in which participants were encouraged to discuss news and current affairs. Working in partnership with Dr. Dan Nightingale over a 9-month period, Duff established that people living with dementia who had been given hypnosis therapy exhibited improved concentration, memory and socialization compared to the other two treatment groups. Relaxation, motivation and daily living activities also improved with the use of hypnosis. (Cf. References, Study 25)

Hypnosis Speeds Wound Healing

In a randomized, controlled trial, 18 healthy women were randomized to one of the three treatments after breast reduction surgery: usual care, additional supportive attention, or additional hypnosis sessions targeting accelerated wound healing. The hypnosis group's objectively observed wound healing (digital imagery and staff blind to groups) was significantly greater than the other two groups, indicating that use of a targeted hypnotic intervention can accelerate postoperative wound healing. (Cf. References, Study 26)

Hypnosis Speeds Fracture Repair

In a study at Mass. General's Dept. of Bone and Joint Disease in Boston, 12 adults with bone fractures were followed for 12 weeks, to measure how hypnosis accelerated their healing. Radiographic results showed dramatically improved healing at 6 weeks in the hypnosis patients. Orthopedic assessments of mobility, strength and need for analgesics showed greater improvement in the hypnosis patients at weeks 1, 3 and 9. The hypnotic intervention included audio taped suggestions to reduce swelling, stimulate tissue growth, and fusion at the injury site, and counteract pain and stress; and imagery rehearsals of greater mobility, enhanced bone strength and recovery of normal activities. (Cf. References, Study 27)

Hypnosis for Burns

"Hypnosis has a part to play in nearly every aspect of burn care, from the initial visit through tubbing and grafting, and finally to rehabilitation. Early hypnosis attenuates the inflammatory response to the injury, limiting the usual progression of the burn from first degree to second degree, or from second to third. Procedural pain can be controlled. Guilt or anger about the accident need to be alleviated, caloric intake can be increased, and active participation in physical therapy can be enhanced."
(Cf. References, Study 28)

Hypnosis and Female Incontinence

Fifty incontinent women with proved detrusor instability completed 12 sessions of hypnosis (symptom removal by direct suggestion and "ego strengthening") over one month.

At the end of the 12 sessions, 29 patients were entirely symptom free, 14 improved, and 7 unchanged. Three months later, cystometry in 44 of the patients showed conversion of the cystometrogram to stability in 22 and a significant improvement in a further 16; only 6 showed no objective improvement. ..."*It is concluded that psychological factors are very important in "idiopathic" detrusor instability and that hypnotherapy is effective for incontinence due to this disorder.*" (Cf. References, Study 29)

Hypnosis and Male Sexual Dysfunction

A study comprised 79 men in whom clinical and laboratory examinations revealed no organic cause for their impotence were treated with testosterone (20 men), trazodone (21 men), hypnosis (20 men), or a placebo (18 men), all of comparable age groupings. Their reported results by interview at 4, 6 and 8 weeks after treatment were verified by interviewing their partners. Conclusion: *"The only treatment superior to placebo seemed to be hypnosis."* (Cf. References, Study 30)

Medical Hypnosis Underutilized

Five case histories demonstrate the dramatic and sometimes unexpected beneficial outcomes of medical hypnosis. *"Hypnosis is suitable for patients with the following medical conditions: chronic headache, chronic back pain, psychogenic weakness or paralysis, chronic constipation, irritable bowel syndrome, panic attacks and phobias."* (Cf. References, Study 31)

Hypnosis Works as General Anesthesia

197 thyroidectomies and 21 cervical explorations for hyperparathyroidism were performed under hypno-sedation and compared to a closely matched population of patients operated on under general anesthesia. All patients having hypno-sedation reported a very pleasant experience, had significantly less postoperative pain, significantly reduced analgesic use, significantly shorter

hospital stay, providing a substantial reduction of the medical care costs. Their postoperative convalescence was significantly improved, and full return to social or professional activity was significantly shortened. (Cf. References, Study 32)

Hypnosis Makes Tinnitus Nuisance into Pleasure

A combination of relaxation and imagery was used to teach an altered perception of their chronic tinnitus to a series of clients, for all of whom medical intervention had proved ineffective. After some training sessions, the hum which had been troubling them became a cue for relaxation and peace. Thus, whenever they became aware of their tinnitus it came to be welcomed where prior to intervention it had been a constant irritant. (Cf. References, Study 33)

Hypnosis Permits Ignoring Tinnitus Noise

32 patients, variously diagnosed as suffering from tinnitus, were treated with hypnosis. Treatment consisted of a 1-hour consultation with the physician followed by 4 weeks of daily home practice while listening to an audio-tape recording of approximately 15 minutes duration. 22 of the patients treated learned in only 1 month to disregard the disturbing noise. (Cf. References, Study 34)

Mind-Body Hypnotic Imagery in the Treatment of Auto-Immune Disorders

A systematic review of the literature on the connection between the brain and the immune system and its clinical implications. It then provides a rational foundation for the role of using hypnosis and imagery to therapeutically influence the immune system. Five case examples are provided with illustrated instructions for clinicians on how hypnosis and imagery may be utilized in the treatment of patients with auto-immune disorders. (Cf. References, Study 36)

Hypnosis: An Alternate Approach to Insomnia

"Insomnia sleep disorders can be divided into primary and secondary types. Primary sleep disorders have an autonomous function in the central nervous system. Secondary sleep disorders can result from causes such as depression, pain, anxiety, lifestyle change, etc. Hypnosis seems to be most effective in dealing with the problems of a secondary nature." (Cf. References, Study 37).

Hypnosis for Nausea and Vomiting in Cancer Chemotherapy

Six randomized controlled trials that evaluated the effectiveness of hypnosis in chemotherapy-induced nausea and vomiting (CINV) were analyzed. The clinical commentaries reported a large positive effect, including statistically significant reductions in anticipatory and CINV. (Cf. References, Study 38)

Other Hypnosis Medical Studies

There are thousands of studies of the medical benefits of hypnosis. The above list is just a sampling for the some of the most common medical issues. If you did not find your medical issue listed above, do your own internet search by typing into a search engine such as Google "medical study of hypnosis for ...(your issue)."

STUDY REFERENCES

Study 1: "Preoperative Instruction for Decreased Bleeding During Spine Surgery," *Anesthesiology* 1986; 65:A245.

Study 2: Kathleen Haralson, *Professional's Guide to Exercise and Medical Conditions*, IDEA Health & *Fitness, 2000*, ISBN=188778117X

Study 3: "The Truth About the Truth: a meta-analytic review of the Truth Effect," *Personality and Social Psychology Review* in May 2010 (14(2):238-57).

Appendix A5. Medical Benefits of Hypnosis

Study 4: "A Randomized Clinical Trial of a Brief Hypnosis Intervention to Control Side Effects in Breast Surgery Patients," *Journal of the National Cancer Institute,* 2007 Sep 99(17):1304-12.

Study 5: usatoday30.usatoday.com/news/health/2005-05-09-prayer-pain_x.htm

Study 6: "Rapid Changes in Histone Deacetylases and Inflammatory Gene Expression in Expert Meditators," *Psychoneuroendocrinology.* 2014 Feb;40: 96–107.

Study 7: Timothy McCall, MD, *Yoga As Medicine,* (See entry for book in complete reference list).

Study 8: "Yoga for Chronic Neck Pain: A Pilot Randomized Controlled Clinical Trial," *Journal of Pain,* 2012 Nov;13(11):1122-30.

Study 9: "Beautiful Art Eases Pain," *University World News,* Oct 5, 2008; Issue No:47, www.universityworldnews.com/article.php? story=20081002145858911

Study 10: "A Dose of Music for Pain Relief," *Society for Neuroscience,* Jan 2013, reported by BrainFacts.org www.brainfacts.org/sensing-thinking-behaving/senses-and-perception/articles/2013/a-dose-of-music-for-pain-relief/

Study 11: Dr. Kevin Berry, TMJ Therapy & Sleep Center of Colorado; www.tmjtherapyandsleepcenter.com/chronic-pain-relief-for-a-song/

Study 12: "A Randomized Trial of Tai Chi for Fibromyalgia," *New England Journal of Medicine.* 2010 Aug 19; 363(8):743-54.

Study 13: "Hypnosis in Contemporary Medicine, "Mayo *Clinic Proceedings* 2005; 80:511-524.

Study 14: "Intensive Therapy: Utilizing Hypnosis in the Treatment of Substance Abuse Disorders," Potter, Greg, *American Journal of Clinical Hypnosis,* Jul 2004.

Study 15: "A Comparative Study of Hypnotherapy and Psychotherapy in the Treatment of Methadone Addicts," *American Journal of Clinical Hypnosis,* 1984; 26(4): 273-9.

Study16: "Hypnosis as an Adjunct to Cognitive-Behavioral Psychotherapy for Obesity: A Meta-Analytic Reappraisal," *Journal Consult Clinical Psychol.* 1996; 64(3):513-516.

Study 17: "How One in Five Give Up Smoking," *Journal of Applied Psychology,* October 1992.

Study 18: "Effect of Guided Imagery on Length of Stay, Pain and Anxiety in Cardiac Surgery Patients," *Journal of Cardiovascular Management* 10;2:22-8 1999

Study 19: "A Randomized Clinical Trial of a Brief Hypnosis Intervention to Control Side Effects in Breast Surgery Patients," *Journal of the National Cancer Institute*, 2007 Sep; 99(17):1304-12.

Study 20: "fMRI Used to Investigate Brain Activity Under Hypnosis for Pain Suppression," *Regional Anesthesia and Pain Medicine*, Nov-Dec 2004.

Study 21: "Controlled Trial of Hypnotherapy in the Treatment of Refractory Fibromyalgia," Netherlands, *Journal of Rheumatology 1991, vol. 18, no1, pp. 72-75*

Study 22: "Hypnosis in Dermatology," *Dermatol.* 2000 Mar;136(3):393-9

Study 23: "The Treatment of Irritable Bowel Syndrome with Hypnotherapy," *Appl Psychophysiol Biofeedback.* 1998 Dec;23(4):219-32

Study 24: "Effect of Preoperative Suggestion on Postoperative Gastro-intestinal Motility," *West J Med* 1993 158;5:488-92

Study 25: "Hypnosis Slows Impacts of Dementia and Improves Quality of Life," (www.liv.ac.uk/researchintelligence/issue36/hypnosis.htm), University of Liverpool Research Intelligence.

Study 26: "Can Medical Hypnosis Accelerate Post-Surgical Wound Healing? Results of a Clinical Trial," *Am J Clin Hypn.* 2003 Apr;45(4):333-51.

Study 27: "Using Hypnosis to Accelerate the Healing of Bone Fractures: A Randomized Controlled Pilot Study," *Alter Ther Health Med.* 1999 Mar; 5(2):67-75

Study 28: "The Use of Hypnosis in the Treatment of Burn Patients," *International Handbook of Clinical Hypnosis,* Online ISBN: 9780470846407; DOI=10.1002/ 0470846402.ch19

Study 29: "Hypnotherapy for Incontinence Caused by the Unstable Detrusor." *Br Med J (Clin Res Ed).* 1982 June 19; 284(6332): 1831–1834.

Study 30: "Efficacy of Testosterone, Trazodone and Hypnotic Suggestion in the Treatment of Non-Organic Male Sexual Dysfunction," Yüzüncü Yil University, Van, Turkey. *Br J Urol.* 1996 Feb;77(2):256-60.

Study 31: "Medical Hypnosis: An Underutilized Treatment Approach," *Permanente Journal,* Fall 2001/Vol. 5, No. 4.

Study 32: "Hypnosis with Conscious Sedation Instead of General Anesthesia? Applications in Cervical Endocrine Surgery," University of Liege, Belgium, *Acta Chir Belg.* 1999 Aug;99(4):151-8.

Study 33: "Cognitive Restructuring: A Technique for the Relief of Chronic Tinnitus," *Australian Journal of Clinical and Experimental Hypnosis,* 10 (1), 27-33.

Study 34: "An Alternative Method of Treating Tinnitus: Relaxation-Hypnotherapy Primarily through the Home Use of a Recorded Audio

Appendix A5. Medical Benefits of Hypnosis

Cassette," *International Journal of Clinical and Experimental Hypnosis,* 31 (2), 90-97.

Study 35: "Successful Aging through Digital Games: Socioemotional Differences between Older Adult Gamers and Non-gamers," *Computers in human Behavior,* 2013 July; (29 (4):1302–6.

Study 36: "Mind-Body Hypnotic Imagery in the Treatment of Auto-Immune Disorders," Moshe S. Torem, *American Journal of Clinical Hypnosis,* 50:2, 157-170, DOI:10.1080/00029157.2007.10401612

Study 37: "Hypnosis: An Alternate Approach to Insomnia," Donald C. Paterson, PMCID: PMC2306547, *Can Fam Physician.* 1982 Apr; 28: 768–770.

Study 38: "Hypnosis for Nausea and Vomiting in Cancer Chemotherapy: a Systematic Review of the Research Evidence," Richardson J, *Eur J Cancer Care (Engl).* 2007 Sep;16(5):402-12

~◻~◻~◻~

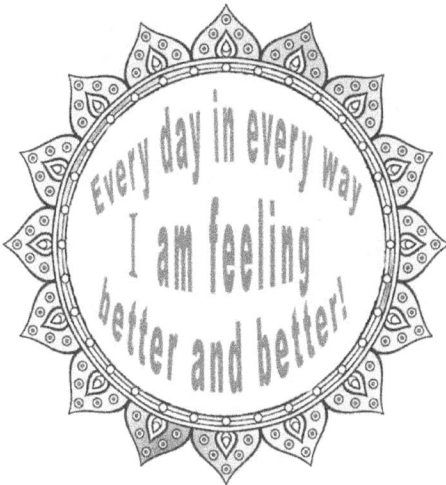

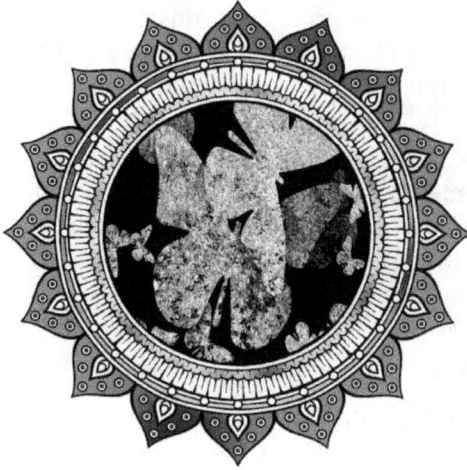

Hypnosis Myths Busted

The Truth in the 11 Worst Hypnosis Myths

There is a saying that every myth has an element of truth in it. Hypnosis is still surrounded by myths in popular culture, and that saying applies to these, my favorites as the worst hypnosis myths. Here are the 11 worst hypnosis myths with the element of *truth* on which they are based, and the *facts* about those myths that bust them.

Myth #1:

Hypnosis is associated with magic, the supernatural, or the work of the devil.

Basis #1: Results of hypnosis appear magical. (My client who came to quit smoking proclaimed this on his second visit: "It's like magic! I haven't had or wanted a cigarette since our session. I don't understand it! How can it be that I am no longer interested in cigarettes?")

Basis #2: Results of hypnosis cannot be adequately explained. What we cannot totally explain by science is often considered *beyond the natural laws* as we understand them, or *supernatural.* (Remember that Galileo Galilei was condemned of heresy by the Inquisition in 1615 for stating that the earth is not at the center of the universe and that it moves around the sun).

Basis #3: Whatever is not understood is often regarded as evil.

Fact: Hypnosis is a natural human state experienced by everyone. It has been extensively studied scientifically. Although we still don't understand much about the mind, we do know how to focus its powers to get results through hypnosis. Hypnotherapy is based on many years of clinical research and documentation by famous psychologists.

Fact: Hypnosis was approved for medical and dental use by the British Medical Association in 1955, by the Pope in 1956, by the American Medical Association in 1958, and endorsed by the American Psychological Association in 1960. Hypnosis is now used in many hospitals. (Hospitals often give hypnosis another name, like visualization or guided imagery, to sidestep this myth).

Myth #2:

A hypnotist is a person who has mysterious or unusual magic-like powers.

Basis: What we don't understand appears magic-like to us.

Fact: A hypnotist does not possess any unusual powers. Hypnotherapists are not psychics, magicians, palm-readers, and do not claim any "special powers." The hypnotist has learned the science and art of effective communication with the subconscious.

Appendix A6. Hypnosis Myths Busted

Fact: Hypnotists know that everyone hypnotizes themselves and that the trance state is a normal part of everyday life. You are entranced by music, by love, by art, by yoga, in meditation, in prayer, and in the boredom of freeway driving. The hypnotist assists you to return to a trance state where you communicate more directly with your inner wisdom to make your desired change.

Fact: Anyone can learn the skills and become a certified hypnotherapist with the proper training. The hypnotist may teach people how to hypnotize themselves whenever they want, as we routinely do at Tooley Hypnosis.

Myth #3:
Hypnosis means being put to sleep or into unconsciousness. It means a loss of control and being *out!*

Basis: Whenever we see a person being very still with their eyes closed, we think they are either asleep or unconscious, and hopefully not dead!

Fact: In hypnosis you are awake in an active state of heightened inner awareness where you can communicate with the hypnotist and continue to make choices and decisions. It is an opportunity to have a conversation with your Higher Self. Because you are so inwardly focused, you relax your muscles with closed eyes and your body is motionless. Therefore, if people see you, they might think that you were asleep or unconscious because that is usually the case when we see someone still with their eyes closed.

Fact: Sometimes a hypnotized person appears to go to sleep. When this happens it is because the person is completely relaxed and wanted or needed to sleep. They still take on the hypnotic suggestions.

Fact: Listening to a hypnosis audio recording at bedtime is a wonderful way to both reinforce your desired change and relax comfortably into sleep. I recommend it. Your subconscious is most receptive as you fall asleep or sleep. See the first or last page of this book for information about hypnosis recordings.

Myth #4:
The hypnotist will be able to control my mind.

Basis #1: In entertainment hypnosis, the volunteers do what the hypnotist instructs, even if it is silly or something they would not ordinarily do.

Basis #2: Mind control continues to be a popular and profitable science fiction theme for entertainment media.

Fact: No one can control your mind, unless you let them (or unless it's your mother!) Your hypnotherapist gives you suggestions that you want based on the information you provide during the interview. You remain free to decide to follow a suggestion or not, whatever you choose.

Myth #5:
I will embarrass myself by revealing something I have kept secret. Hypnosis can get someone to confess.

Basis: "The silly actions of volunteers in entertainment hypnosis seem embarrassing. If they do those embarrassing things under hypnosis, maybe I will too!"

Fact: Hypnosis for therapy is not hypnosis for entertainment. You will only speak about what is necessary to resolve the issue that you have chosen for hypnosis resolution. Your therapist doesn't care what you may have done, and furthermore, is bound to keep it confidential. Your hypnotherapist is only there to help you achieve what you want, and has probably heard it all before anyway. With hypnosis, you can resolve an issue by admitting to yourself its source without telling the details to the hypnotist. The hypnotist's role is to hold a mirror so that you can see yourself (and your own inner wisdom) more clearly.

Myth #6:
A person in a hypnotic state may not be easily awakened and may remain in that state for a long time. Hypnosis is a dangerous experience.

Basis: Speculation that a hypnotized person is in a very deep, comatose state and that the action of a hypnotist is necessary to bring a person out of that state.

Fact: Awakened is not the proper term, because the person was never asleep. The hypnotist knows and uses the correct method to bring a person back from a trance state to *normal room awareness* at the end of the session. Even if this were not done, the hypnotized person will exit the hypnosis state naturally when ready.

Fact: There is no historical record of anyone ever failing to emerge from a hypnotic state!

Fact: As part of your self-hypnosis training, you will learn both how to put yourself into a trance and how to bring yourself out of a trance whenever you want. Hypnosis is very safe and is in fact, a state of hyper-awareness. My clients report hearing every little sound, but are able to ignore them. If there were an emergency, you would be able to come out of the hypnotic state naturally by opening your eyes and stretching or speaking.

Myth #7:
I can't be hypnotized because my mind is too strong and disciplined.

Basis: Some people report that they tried hypnosis and they were not hypnotized.

Fact: Because hypnosis is such a natural, familiar state, many people who are successfully hypnotized do not think they were hypnotized until they experience the results that they programmed themselves to achieve under hypnosis. Many of my clients tell me later that they didn't think anything happened until they experienced their desired change in their life.

Fact: Because hypnosis accomplishes change in the subconscious without active participation of the conscious mind, the conscious mind afterward is often unaware of the changes as they take place. I have had clients who did not notice that their life had dramatically changed because it felt so familiar, natural, and effortless. They became aware that what they had programmed under hypnosis was now occurring in their life only when a friend or family member called their attention to their changed behavior. Conscious willpower was not required because their subconscious easily implemented their desired adjustment.

Fact: There is a spectrum of ease of going into hypnosis. Some people hypnotize themselves more easily than others. If you can follow directions and are willing to be hypnotized, you CAN be hypnotized. Even if you are at the more difficult end of the spectrum, you can still be hypnotized; the hypnotist just has to work a little more at getting you hypnotized. (I monitor the external signs of hypnosis in my clients to determine when they go into a trance and continue to use appropriate hypnosis-inducing language until they do so.)

Fact: Hypnosis is a learned skill. You can learn to hypnotize yourself easily and accomplish many of the changes that you desire. I teach my clients how to use self-hypnosis to achieve their goals.

Myth #8:

I have never been hypnotized before.

Basis: You have never seen a hypnotist or hypnotherapist.

Fact: Every person naturally enters a state of hypnosis at least twice every day: just before falling asleep at night, and upon awaking every morning before getting out of bed. Formal hypnosis simply duplicates the relaxed, partly drowsy, highly-suggestible state of those two times.

Fact: Most people easily enter a state of *environment hypnosis* while at the movies, watching TV, driving on the highway, or reading a good book.

Fact: You were probably hypnotized by your parents for your first few years of childhood (until you figured out how to hypnotize them!)

Fact: If you are an athlete, you experience hypnosis as *getting into the zone.*

Fact: If you have ever been in love, you experienced the ultimate hypnotic state!

Myth #9:

After hypnosis, I will have no memory of the session and won't know what happened.

Basis: You don't remember things from when you are asleep or unconscious.

Fact: Hypnosis is not an unconscious state or sleep. In fact, most people report having a heightened sense of awareness, concentration, and focus. You will have a conversation with me as your hypnotist during the session. I will instruct you to remember everything. You will get some reminders of the session to take home with you as reinforcements afterward.

Myth #10:
Hypnosis is not effective or takes a lot of expensive sessions.

Basis: Many types of therapy take a lot of sessions, so hypnosis must take many sessions too.

Fact: Hypnosis is very effective. Many hospitals use some form of hypnosis to prepare patients for surgery and assist their rapid recovery. Hypnosis is *THE* most effective method of releasing the tobacco habit.

Fact: Some issues can be solved with a single hypnosis session reinforced by personal self-hypnosis. More deeply entrenched issues take a few sessions.

Fact: Here is the hypnosis effectiveness statistics, results of a comparative study published in American Health Magazine:

- *Psychoanalysis therapy* has, on average, 38% recovery after 600 sessions.
- *Behavior therapy* has, on average, 72% recovery after 22 sessions.
- *Hypnotherapy* has, on average, 93% recovery after 6 sessions.

> *(Statistics gathered by Dr. Alfred Barrios, PhD and documented at: www.stresscards.com/hypnotherapy_reappraisal.php)*

Myth #11:
I will do embarrassing things, such as imitate a dog, chicken, or duck.

Basis: Observing entertainment hypnosis where the volunteers do these things when instructed by the hypnotist.

Fact: This myth results from confusion of therapeutic clinical hypnosis with entertainment hypnosis (stage hypnosis). Stage hypnosis follows a fixed format for entertainment.

Here is how stage hypnosis for entertainment works:

1. A stage hypnotist is hired to entertain a group.
2. The hypnotist asks for volunteers who want to be hypnotized.
3. Volunteers from the group come up on stage. Most of them are just curious.
4. By volunteering, they have made a tacit agreement with the hypnotist: "We are going to have fun doing whatever you say, even being silly!" They know that they can always blame anything they feel embarrassed about afterward on the hypnotist.
5. Often one or more of the volunteers has a different agenda, namely, to *bust* the hypnotist and prove that hypnosis is a fake. (I call them the *disrupters)*.
6. The hypnotist's first task is to sort out these disrupters and tell them to go sit back in the audience. (If you have seen a stage show, you may remember seeing the hypnotist send someone off the stage).
7. The hypnotist then hypnotizes the volunteers.
8. The hypnotist gives them some silly things to do and they do them (to varying degrees).
9. Those hypnotized have a choice to accept or reject the suggestions to act like a chicken or dog, and many accept them! (Perhaps they will deny their choice later because of embarrassment or some other reason).
10. The hypnotist may tell people to be "rigid as a piece of steel" and then support them horizontally by only head and heels. (This demonstrates the extreme power of your subconscious mind over your body because staying stiff horizontally is something you cannot do consciously!)
11. The hypnotist may give a temporary post-hypnotic suggestion, such as "You will forget the number 3."
12. The hypnotist brings the individual out of trance and has them count the fingers on their hand. Invariably they will say: "1, 2, 4, 5, 6," and be totally confused about how they got 6 fingers on that hand,

13. Alternatively, the hypnotist may instruct a person to "Jump up and cheer whenever I say *blue.*"

14. During a conversation, when the hypnotist casually says *blue* the person involuntarily jumps up and cheers but doesn't really understand why he did it. Some inner impulse just caused him to do it.

15. Everybody laughs and has fun, and the awesome power behind hypnosis is revealed as available for therapeutic or performance use.

Fact: Entertainment is never part of therapeutic hypnosis, which is a serious process of self-improvement. Understanding aspects of how entertainment hypnosis works is useful because the powerful aspects of hypnosis that are used in stage hypnosis are equally available for therapeutic and performance hypnosis:

Fact: You accept suggestions more easily when hypnotized.

Fact: Your subconscious has powerful control over your body and can demonstrate that control in hypnosis. (It has that same control at all times. That is why medical hypnosis is so powerful. Giving your subconscious instructions to repair and restore your body will accelerate healing.)

Fact: Post-hypnotic suggestions work automatically without thought because they come from the subconscious.

Conclusion: HYPNOSIS MYTHS BUSTED!

Now that you know better, utilize the safe power of hypnosis to get the life that you want. You can banish discomfort, repair your body, eliminate illness, add skills, drop useless habits and increase your performance and joy. See the products page at the back of the book or go to *store.DuncanTooley.com* for more information.

Still have questions about hypnosis?

Call me at *310-832-0830* or send an email to me at: *Duncan @ DuncanTooley.com*

~☐~☐~☐~

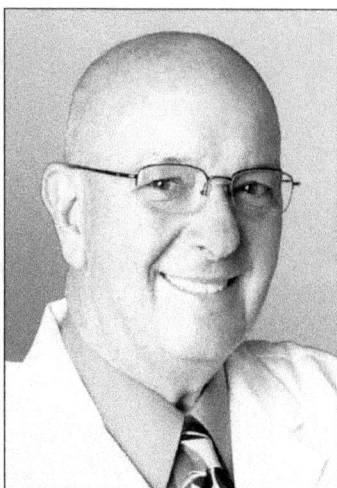

ABOUT THE AUTHOR

Duncan Tooley is a mind trainer, medical hypnotherapist, artist, author, speaker, and life coach. He teaches others to change their thinking, beliefs, and habits. This results in pain-free, lower-weight, less-stressed clients feeling themselves more in control of their health and emotions.

As a Catholic religious bother, Duncan taught high school science for 7 years before beginning his 35-year secular career in corporate information technology interrupted by disabling neuropathy. After years of ineffective medical treatment, he discovered hypnosis and used it to clear his illness. This transformation, and its accompanying spiritual awakening, inspired his career change to become a mind trainer, medical hypnotist, and coach specializing in weight reduction and pain relief. (See his story in the Preface).

Duncan is a lifelong artist, creator of a unique hypnotic weight loss program, Toastmasters International speaker, presenter to cancer support organizations, and Certified Hypnosis Instructor (CHI) for the International Hypnosis Federation.

Do-It-Yourself Pain Relief Resources
You Deserve to Feel GREAT!
I know you can easily adjust to feel great!

Additional tools available at:
feelgreat.duncantooley.com

- Mantra Reminder Cards
- Tooley 60-Second Turn Down Process
- Acupressure Tapping Points Diagram
- Tune Your Mindset Worksheet
- My Comfort Control Chart
- Positive Words That Will Enrich Your Mind & Soul
- Positive Affirmation List
- Feel Great Word Search Puzzle
- List of Medical Issues Benefiting from Hypnosis
- Sunrise Mandala Image
- Mandala Coloring Book

Email Contact: *duncan@duncantooley.com*
Call **310-832-0830 for hypnosis at-a-distance options**
Also see artworks by the author at: **art.duncantooley.com.***com,*
and more hypnosis information at: *hypnosis.duncantooley.com*

www.ingramcontent.com/pod-product-compliance
Lightning Source LLC
Chambersburg PA
CBHW060520280326
41933CB00014B/3037